FIBROIDS

What Every Woman Should Know About this Uterine Foe

By

Myron E. Moorehead, M.D.
Bryan A. Lewis, Ph.D.

First published by AuthorHouse 09/04/04

ISBN: 1-4184-6087-7 (e-book)
ISBN: 1-4184-4461-8 (Paperback)

This book is printed on acid free paper.

TABLE OF CONTENTS

TO THE READER

We know that by obtaining this book you want clear and relevant information about fibroids. We hope to provide that for you. We are not going to bore you with detailed medical jargon which may be intimidating, confusing, or just incomprehensible. Knowledge is power and it is our sincere wish that you are empowered by the information presented in this guide. Only then can you make the right decision for yourself.

FEAR OF THE UNKNOWN

Fear of the unknown can cause anguish, anxiety, depression and other types of debilitating emotions. This will cause both a drain on you emotionally and physically. We hope to prevent you from experiencing these negative pressures so....

FIRST,

Fibroids are not cancerous. Thus, this is not the big "C". Although they are called fibroid tumors they are not cancerous. However, cancerous tumors can occur in the uterus and can be confused with the appearance of a fibroid.

SECOND,

Fibroids can be effectively treated and with the patient being fully informed the treatment option is up to YOU!

Now, that we have this important information out of the way, let's learn something about fibroids so that you can begin that important step of self-empowerment. Don't let anyone take that away from you.

FIBROID: THE UTERINE FOE

We all know what a foe is. It is an enemy or opponent. In this sense, fibroids can be considered enemies of the uterus. When present they can cause a range of disturbing symptoms or none at all. However, if they are present, there is the potential for them to cause symptoms.

Some women have fibroids but are fortunate enough not to have them cause any symptoms or problems. But sadly, many women with these tumors are not this lucky and need medical treatment.

The types of medical treatment options will be discussed later but for now we would like to offer a perspective. In the context of a fibroid being a foe let's look at an analogy. Let's say your uterus is your home and the fibroid is a foe or unwanted visitor in your home causing problems. What do you do, remove the foe or destroy your home? Who would burn down or demolish their home if they could simply remove the foe. Keep this in mind when considering your treatment choices. If the fibroid(s) can be safely removed why remove an entire pelvic organ? But, remember, the choice is **YOURS**. This is your organ, not the physician's.

SOME GENERAL BACKGROUND ON FIBROIDS

JUST WHAT ARE FIBROIDS?

Fibroids, or fibroid tumors, are the most common benign (non-cancerous) tumors (abnormal mass of tissue) of the uterus in the female reproductive system. These benign growths develop from the smooth muscle layer of the uterus.

THERE ARE OTHER NAMES FOR FIBROIDS

Other names for fibroids or fibroid tumors include:

- leiomyomata (lie-o-mi-o-ma-ta)
- leiomyomas (lie-o-mi-o-mas)
- myomas (mie-o-mas)
- fibromyomas (fi-bro-mie-o-mas)
- fibromas (fi-bro-mas)

DO FIBROIDS LEAD TO CANCER?

NO. Fibroids do not become cancerous growths. Lets repeat it. Fibroids are not cancerous growths. People confuse fibroids and cancer because a fibroid is a tumor. But, fibroids are benign tumors.

WHAT ARE THE SIZES OF FIBROIDS?

Fibroids can be the size of a pea or smaller but can grow to the size of a cantaloupe or larger. So, there is considerable variation in their size range.

WHAT DO FIBROIDS LOOK LIKE?

Fibroids have spherical, oblong, or irregular shapes and may cause the uterus to become enlarged and irregular.

THE ORIGIN OF FIBROIDS

The exact cause(s) for the formation of fibroids is unknown. It is suggested that genetic factors may play a role and this mechanism is currently being investigated. It appears that there is an error in the gene that controls the replication rate of uterine muscle cells. Fibroids are more common in African American women than any other ethnic group therefore, suggesting a genetic correlation. Fibroids feed on the hormone estrogen and grow in response to this body chemical. Thus, they tend to grow until menopause from which they tend to shrink because the body ceases producing this hormone. We will return to this discussion later after some background on the female reproductive cycle.

HOW FIBROIDS DEVELOP

Fibroids are the result of accelerated growth of uterine muscle cells. The cells subsequently increase in number and form a compact mass known as the fibroid tumor or simply, fibroid.

HOW LARGE DO FIBROIDS HAVE TO BE BEFORE THEY CAUSE SYMPTOMS?

This question is difficult to answer because symptoms caused by fibroids depend on several factors. It depends on their location and presenting symptoms: Example – Submucus fibroids are located in the uterine cavity and will cause heavy bleeding and anemia. Subserosal fibroids can be large and produce pressure in the pelvic area, or put pressure on other structures.

FIBROIDS: WHO GETS THEM? WHY ME?

No one knows why some women develop fibroids and others do not. However, some women may have fibroids but are unaware that they are present unless they cause symptoms. For this reason, we cannot determine the number of women who have these benign tumors…but estimates are >50%. Heredity may be a factor and the uterine muscle cells may be programmed to develop into a fibroid prior to birth.

DO FIBROIDS OCCUR IN ANY PARTICULAR AGE GROUP?

Fibroids can occur in females from age of 16 to over 50 years of age. The tumors most often develop between the ages of 30 and 40, but rarely occur after menopause. Also they seldom develop before the age of 20. There appears to be a relationship between fibroid growth and estrogen dominant cycles.

ETHNICITY (RACE) AND FIBROIDS

Fibroids can be found in the uterus of women of all ethnic groups but they are more common in African-American women. It is not known why African-American women have a higher incidence of fibroids with an occurrence rate two to five times more often than in white women.

IMPACT OF FIBROIDS ON GYNECOLOGIC SURGERY

The impact of fibroids on gynecologic surgery is significant. Fibroids have contributed to the increase in number of women undergoing hysterectomies in the United States. This book will provide information about alternatives to hysterectomies for fibroids. Approximately 600,000 hysterectomies are performed per year in the U.S. and 1/3 to 1/2 are performed because of uterine fibroids.

HOW MANY FIBROIDS GROW IN THE UTERUS?

Fibroids vary greatly in number from one woman to another so there is no set number that can be found in a given uterus. However, African American women have a greater number of fibroids present than other ethnic women.

THE FEMALE REPRODUCTIVE SYSTEM

AN OVERVIEW

UNDERSTANDING THE FEMALE REPRODUCTIVE SYSTEM

Since fibroids are found in the uterus and their growth is dependent on hormones, it becomes necessary to provide some background on anatomy and physiology of the female reproductive system. It will make the understanding of fibroid treatment and management easier later on.

COMPONENTS OF THE SYSTEM

The female reproductive system consists of the **ovaries, fallopian tubes, uterus**, and **vagina**. In addition to these organs, the mammary glands are also considered part of the female reproductive system.

THE OVARIES

Location of the Ovaries

The ovaries (o-va-rees), also called **gonads** (go-nads), are two almond-shaped glands that lie on each side of the uterus. Glands are organs that secrete substances in the body.

Function of the Ovaries

The function of the ovaries is to produce and release an ovum or egg and insure its survival for possible fertilization by the male's sperm. Ovaries are also responsible for the production of eggs and the secretion of the female hormones **estrogen** (es-tro-gen) and **progesterone** (pro-ges-te-rone).

Menstruation vs Fertilization (Pregnancy)

A fertilized egg must attach to the endometrium which is the inner lining of the uterus. The ovaries produce estrogen and progesterone that causes the endometrium to thicken so that it can support a fertilized egg. If the egg is not fertilized, the thick endometrium lining is not needed so it is shed in the process of menstruation. If the egg is fertilized, the woman is pregnant and the thick lining is able to support products of conception (i.e. placenta and fetus)

FALLOPIAN TUBES

The fallopian (fah-lo-pee-un) tubes are tubes that extend from the ovaries to the uterus. One main function is to transport the egg from the ovary to the uterus. Inside the fallopian tube is also where sperm can meet and fertilize the egg.

UTERUS

The uterus (yoo-ter-us), also called the **womb**, is a pear-shaped, hollow, thick-walled organ that is situated between the urinary bladder and the rectum. The uterus serves multiple functions such as:

- the site where a fertilized egg implants itself
- the organ in which a fetus develops during pregnancy
- avenue in which sperm can reach the fallopian tubes
- site of menstruation

Since the uterus is the target organ for fibroids, we will provide a full discussion of this organ later.

VAGINA

The vagina is a tubular muscular organ that lies between the urinary bladder and the rectum. Because the vagina serves as the passageway for delivery of an infant, it is also referred to as the birth canal. The vagina also provides a passageway for the flow of menses from the uterus and it receives the penis and semen during sexual intercourse.

THE UTERUS: SITE OF THE FIBROIDS

ANATOMY OF THE UTERUS

The uterus is structurally divided into three main parts called the **fundus**, the **body**, and the **cervix (ser-viks)**.

1. The fundus is the top portion of the uterus that is relatively wide and dome-shaped.

2. The body is the central portion of the uterus and,

3. The cervix is the bottom narrow portion that opens into the vagina.

The interior portion of the uterus is called the uterine cavity.

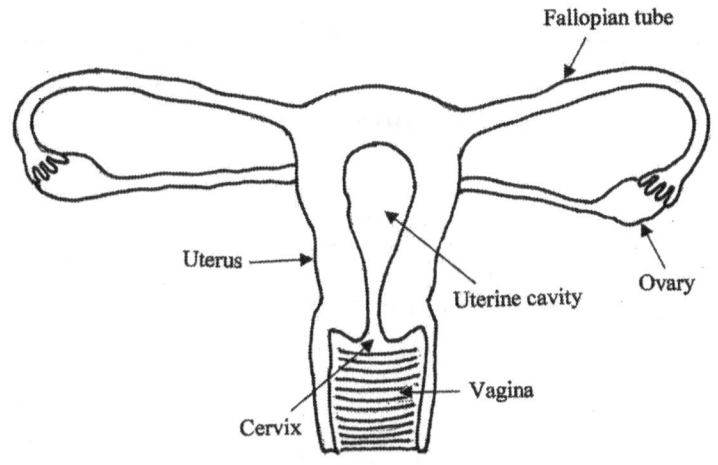

THE TISSUES OF THE UTERUS

There are three layers of tissue found in the uterus which are the

1) **perimetrium** (pe-ree-mee-tri-um),
2) **myometrium** (mi-o-mee-tri-um), and the
3) **endometrium** (en-do-mee-tri-um).

The perimetrium is the outer layer and the myometrium is the middle or muscle layer that forms the bulk of the uterine wall. The endometrium is the inner layer of the uterus and it is subdivided into two layers. One layer is closest to the myometrium and the other layer is closer to the uterine cavity.

7

The layer closest to the uterine cavity is the one that is shed during menstruation. After this layer is shed, more is produced by the underlying layer that is closest to the myometrium.

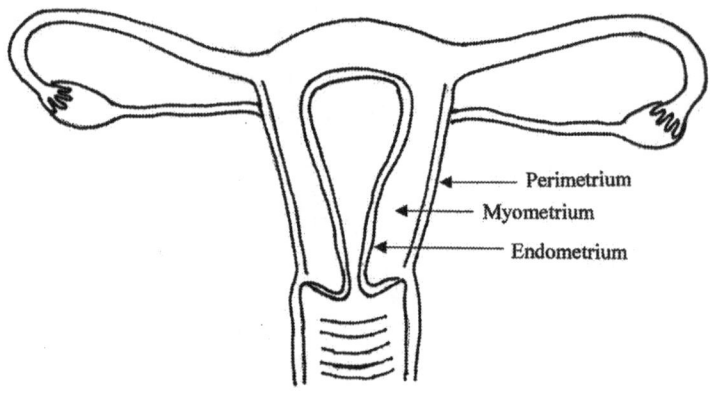

Perimetrium

Myometrium

Endometrium

UNDERSTANDING THE FEMALE REPRODUCTIVE CYCLE

THE TWO REPRODUCTIVE CYCLES

The female reproductive cycle consists of two cycles called:
1) the **ovarian cycle** and the
2) **uterine (menstrual) cycle**.

FUNCTIONS OF THE REPRODUCTIVE CYCLES

The ovarian cycle

The ovarian cycle is responsible for the production of a mature egg in the ovary

The uterine cycle

The uterine cycle is responsible for cyclic changes that the uterus undergoes each month resulting in periods.

Both of these cycles are controlled by regulatory chemicals called **hormones.** Before we begin a brief discussion on the female reproductive cycles, we need to provide a background on hormones to understand how these cycles work and how hormonal therapy can be used to treat fibroids.

HORMONES

THE ROLE OF HORMONES

The human body is made up of many cells and is therefore called a **multicellular** organism. In order for all of the component parts of the body to work together, there must be some type of regulation of the different components. To achieve this, the function of certain cells can be controlled and regulated by chemicals called **hormones**. Thus, hormones are **regulatory chemicals**.

WHERE ARE HORMONES PRODUCED?

Hormones are produced in glands called **endocrine** (en'-do-krin) **glands**. A gland consists of cells that produce and secrete a specific product.

THE PRODUCTION OF THE FEMALE HORMONES

The ovaries (or gonads) are glands that secrete estrogen and progesterone (reproductive hormones). The ovaries also contain the eggs and with hormone stimulation from the pituitary these eggs will mature and ovulation occurs. We will expand on this.

WHAT HAPPENS TO HORMONES PRODUCED BY THE GLANDS?

An endocrine gland produces and secretes its hormones into the bloodstream where it only binds to specific cells called **target cells**. This means that a hormone will travel throughout the body but it knows which cell it is supposed to affect. It's like walking down a hall with many doors but you know which door to enter.

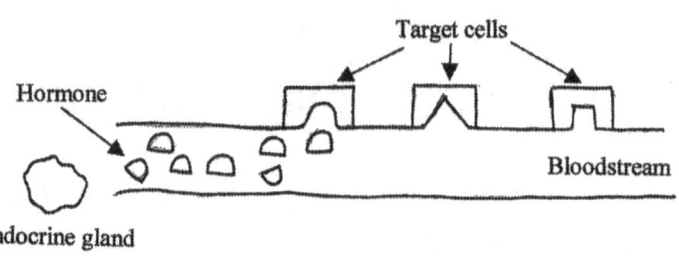

HOW DOES A HORMONE KNOW ITS TARGET CELL?

The target cell for a specific hormone has specific binding sites for that hormone that is called **receptors**. It is through these receptors that the hormone recognizes its target cells. We can think of the hormone as being a key and its target cell as a door that has several locks (receptors) that recognize the particular key.

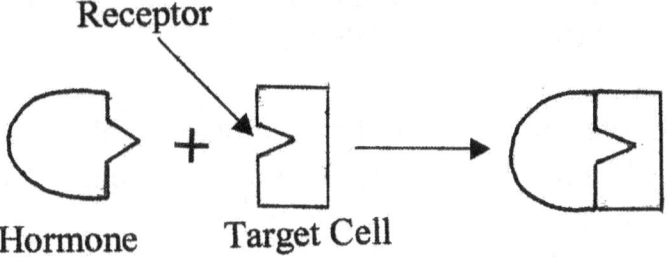

THE FEMALE HORMONES

HORMONES INVOLVED IN THE FEMALE REPRODUCTIVE CYCLE.

The role and action of the hormones involved in the female reproductive cycle will be discussed later but, for now we will simply list them.

- Gonadotropin (go-nad-o-tro-pin) releasing hormone (**GnRH)**

- Follicle-stimulating hormone (**FSH)**

- Luteinizing (loo-tee-in-iz-ing) hormone (**LH)**

- Estrogen (es-tro-gen)

- Progesterone (pro-ges-te-rone)

WHERE ARE THE FEMALE HORMONES LOCATED?

THE HYPOTHALAMUS

The hypothalamus (hi-po-thal-ah-mus) is a small region of the brain that produces hormones that control the function of the **gonads**, which are the **ovaries** in females and testes in males.

The hormones produced by the hypothalamus are called gonadotropin (go-nad-o-tro-pin) releasing hormones (GnRH) and their target site is the anterior pituitary gland.

GNRH

HYPOTHALAMUS ⟹ **ANTERIOR PITUITARY**

(TARGET)

THE PITUITARY GLAND

The pituitary (pi-too-i-tae-ree) gland is a small pea-size gland also found in the brain that has two structural portions called the **anterior** and **posterior** portion.

The anterior pituitary gland produces and secretes two hormones called **gonadotropins** because they regulate and control the function of the gonads (ie. ovaries). The two gonadotropins produced are the **follicle-stimulating hormone (FSH)** and the **luteinizing hormone (LH)**.

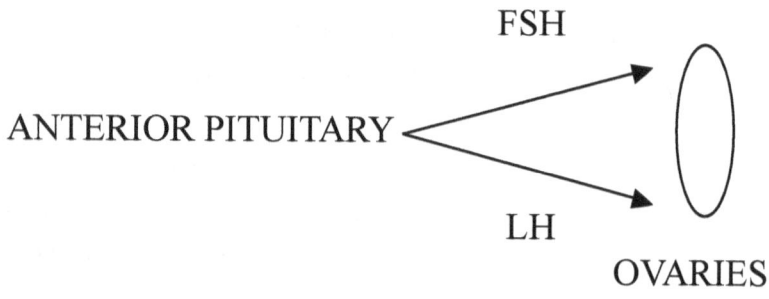

THE OVARIES

The follicles in the ovaries secrete the hormone estrogen once they are stimulated by FSH from the anterior pituitary gland. Also, progesterone is produced during ovulation. This will be described in the next section. The follicles also house the oocytes or eggs.

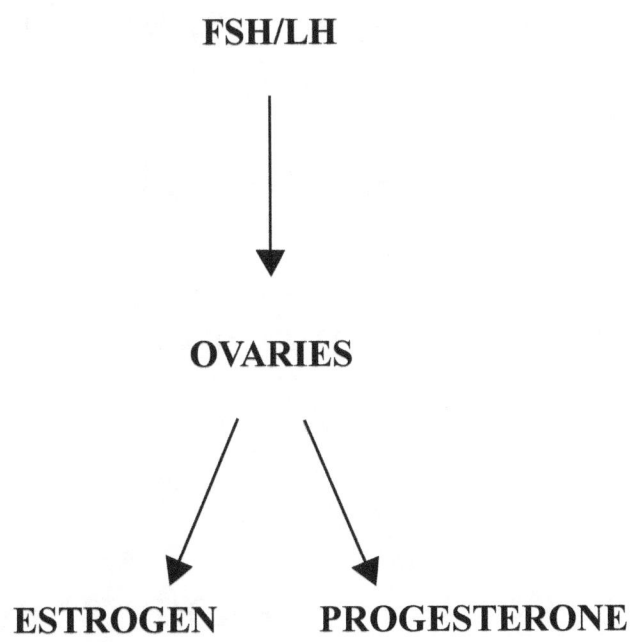

FSH/LH

OVARIES

ESTROGEN   **PROGESTERONE**

THE BIG PICTURE OF HORMONAL REGULATION

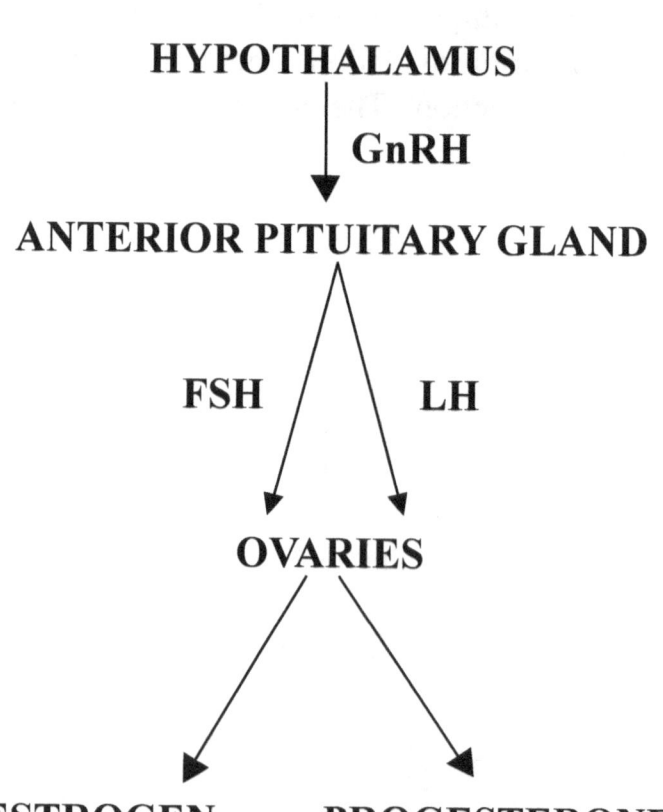

HYPOTHALAMUS

GnRH

ANTERIOR PITUITARY GLAND

FSH   LH

OVARIES

ESTROGEN   PROGESTERONE

Elevated levels of estrogen circulating in the blood can inhibit both the release of GnRH by the hypothalamus and FSH and LH by the anterior pituitary

THE OVARIAN CYCLE

The Ovaries and Egg Production

When a human female is born she has about 700,000 immature eggs called **oocytes** (o-o-sites) in each of her ovaries. However, by the time she reaches sexual maturity, she has about 200,000 oocytes due to the process of degeneration.

The Function of the Ovarian Cycle

The ovaries in a fertile female will go through a monthly ovarian cycle in which only one oocyte will form into a mature egg called an **ovum** that is released during each cycle (period).

The Ovaries Alternate in Egg Production

The ovaries alternate in the production of one ovum each month. This means that one ovary produces an ovum one month and the other ovary produces an ovum the next month.

During a woman's life, oocytes are constantly degenerating but no replacements are being formed. Thus, at menopause a woman will have only a few oocytes remaining in each ovary.

Egg Development in the Ovaries

The ovaries contain numerous tiny spherical chambers called **follicles** in which the oocytes are found. Each follicle, which consists of one or more layers of cells, contains an oocyte.

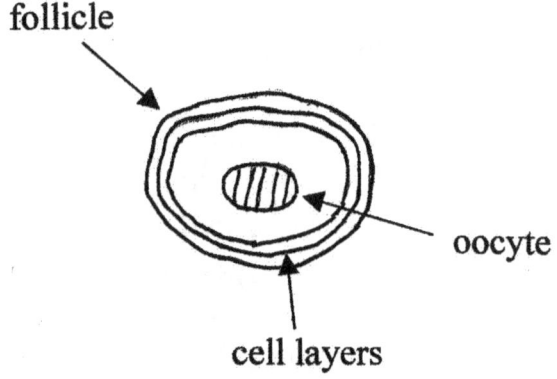

follicle

oocyte

cell layers

Once these cells are stimulated by **the follicle-stimulating hormone (FSH)**, they begin to produce the hormone **estrogen**. Estrogen causes the growth and development of the follicles, but only one develops into a mature follicle called the **Graafian follicle**.

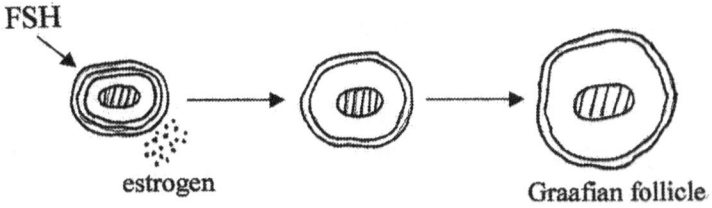

Ovulation

Ovulation is the process by which the Graafian follicle ruptures and releases the mature egg or ovum. This rupture is caused by a hormone called the **luteinizing hormone (LH)**.

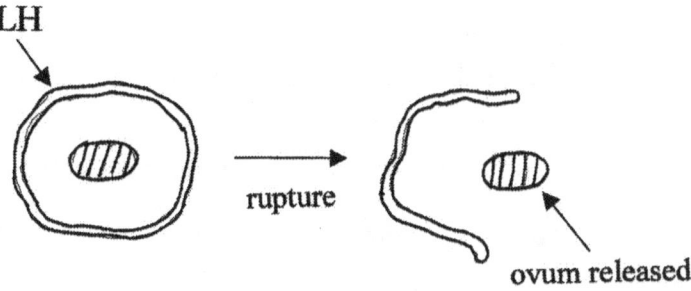

The remainder of the Graafian follicle reforms into a gland called the **corpus luteum** which begins to produce the hormones estrogen and progesterone. The progesterone in conjunction with estrogen is responsible for preparing the uterine lining (endometrium) to receive a fertilized egg.

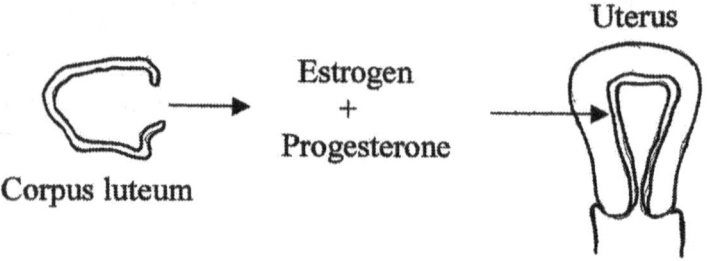

Corpus luteum → Estrogen + Progesterone → Uterus

Pregnancy vs Nonpregnancy

If an egg is fertilized, it travels to the uterus where it specifically attaches to the endometrium and the woman is now pregnant. However, if an egg is not fertilized, the endometrium breaks down and, both it and the unfertilized egg, are discharged through the vagina in the process known as menstruation.

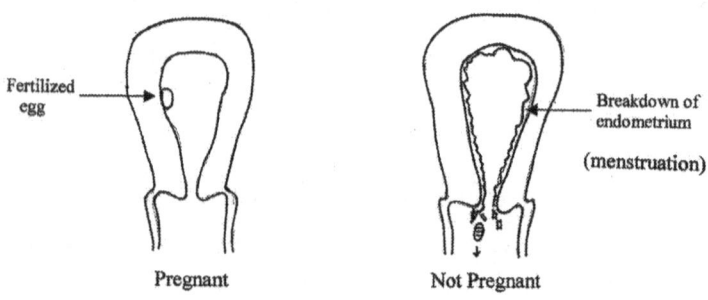

Fertilized egg — Pregnant

Breakdown of endometrium (menstruation) — Not Pregnant

THE UTERINE (MENSTRUAL) CYCLE

The menstrual cycle is a series of changes that the endometrium of the uterus undergoes during monthly cycles. The continual repair and breakdown of the endometrium (menstruation) occurs because of changes in the levels of estrogen and progesterone that are released during the ovarian cycle.

MANAGEMENT OF
FIBROIDS

DIAGNOSIS OF FIBROIDS

Since a large number of women who have fibroids never experience symptoms (they are asymptomatic), they are usually diagnosed when their physician performs a pelvic examination. After a pelvic exam, the physician can confirm the diagnosis of suspected fibroids by using several diagnostic procedures.

Pelvic Examination

The pelvic examination done by the physician is called a bimanual examination. In the examination the physician places two fingers in the vagina and places the other hand on the surface of the abdomen. The cervix is then elevated with the two fingers to position it close to the wall of the abdomen. Then, by pressing down on the abdomen with the other hand, the size and physical shape of the uterus can be ascertained.

Ultrasonography (Ultrasound)

Ultrasound is a technology in which reflected sound waves are used to create an image of the uterus and other pelvic organs. The images are projected onto a monitor. It is a very accurate diagnostic procedure for fibroids and can detect their numbers, sizes, and location. In the abdominal ultrasound (transabdominal) procedure, a device that resembles a computer mouse is rubbed across the abdomen after cream is applied to the area to make it easier to glide. The vaginal ultrasound (transvaginal) procedure uses a wand-like probe that is inserted into the vagina from which the images are generated. The ultrasound is the least expensive procedure and will always suffice to make the diagnosis and support the method of treatment.

Magnetic Resonance Imaging (MRI)

Magnetic resonance imaging (MRI) is an imaging technique used to produce high quality images of component parts inside of the human body. It uses a powerful magnetic field and radio signals to generate detailed images of the uterus, fallopian tubes, and ovaries. The MRI procedure is performed by having the woman lie motionless on a cushion while the machine takes the picture. The patient must remove all metal objects before beginning the procedure.

CT SCAN (CAT SCAN)

The CT or CAT scan stands for computed axial tomography. The CT scan procedure uses x-rays and computers to produce images of soft body tissues. However, the role of CT scans is limited in the diagnosis of fibroids. Both CT scan and MRI procedures are much more expensive than ultrasound.

Hysterosalpingogram (HSG)

Hysterosalpingogram is an x-ray procedure used to examine abnormal changes in the size and shape of the uterus. However, HSG is most often used to determine blockage in the fallopian tubes.

Diagnostic Hysteroscopy

In this procedure, a tube-like instrument called a hysteroscope is inserted through the vagina and cervix. This scope has a light and camera system which allows the physician to see inside of the uterus cavity and locate a submucus fibroid.

Diagnostic Laparoscopy

In this procedure a tube-like instrument called a laparoscope is inserted through the navel into the abdomen. The uterus can be visualized and determined if it is enlarged or contains a intramural or subserosal fibroid.

WHERE ARE FIBROIDS LOCATED?

Fibroids can be located at various sites in the uterus and their particular location can have a major influence on the symptoms produced. Fibroids are classified by their location in the uterus and include the following:

- Intramural
- Submucosal
- Subserosal
- Pedunculated

Submucosal or intracavitary fibroids can be associated with recurrent pregnancy loss, infertility, heavy bleeding and anemia.

Subserosal or intramural fibroids located in the wall of the uterus can cause the uterus to be very large and irregular.

Fibroids found in the inner cavity or muscle wall of the uterus may cause menstrual cramping and painful menstruation called dysmenorrhea.

Pedunculated fibroids are fibroids that grow on stalks called peduncles. These type of fibroids can be located in the cavity of the uterus or located growing from the surface of the uterus. They are often confused with an enlarged ovary or ovarian tumor.

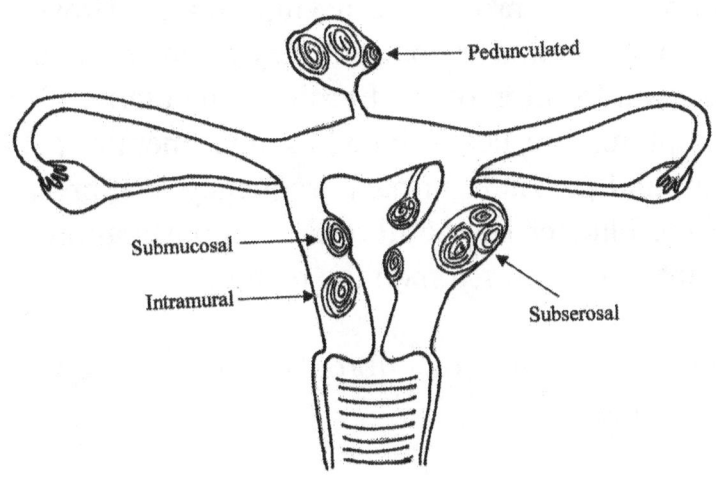

SYMPTOMS OF FIBROIDS

It is well known that many women are unaware that they have uterine fibroids, concluding that in many cases fibroids are asymptomatic. However, when symptoms are present they often relate to the size and location of the fibroid in the uterus. These symptoms are heavy bleeding and anemia, pelvic pain and pressure, urinary frequency, compression of the bladder by the fibroid and constipation as a result of compression on the rectum.

The symptoms of fibroids can include the following:

- Abnormal bleeding
- heavy menstrual bleeding with clotting
- bleeding between periods
- Anemia
- Severe, prolonged abdominal pain
- Frequent urge to urinate
- Backache
- Constipation
- Uterine cramping
- Abdominal enlargement

- Infertility
- Recurrent miscarriages
- Painful intercourse

SUSPECTED CAUSES OF FIBROID DEVELOPMENT

Little is known about the cause of fibroids or what may trigger their growth. Factors causing fibroids could be genetic, hormonal, environmental or, any or all of these in combination.

ESTROGEN PRODUCTION

It is known that in the presence of increased estrogen levels, fibroids are stimulated to increase in size and, in the presence of low estrogen levels fibroids decrease in size. It is also suggested that these are estrogen-like substances in our environment that once introduced into the human body can have estrogen-like affects on fibroid growth and development.

HORMONAL CHANGES

There is thought to be certain 5 time periods in a woman's reproductive years where there are hormonal changes that could account for fibroid stimulation. These are periods of estrogen dominance.

Puberty

Puberty is a time early in life when the pituitary-ovarian hormonal cycle is not yet synchronized thereby producing cycles of estrogen dominance. This increased estrogen environment may well trigger a mechanism for the formation of fibroid tumors.

Pregnancy

Pregnancy is a nine-month period when estrogen, progesterone or other hormones are excessively produced and give rise to rapid growth of uterine fibroids. Also, by 8 weeks postpartum many of the fibroids have significantly decreased in size. This increased/decreased hormonal phenomenon suggests that fibroid growth is dependent upon these changes.

Obesity

Obesity is a common association with fibroids in the reproductive years of women. Again this condition produces an estrogen dominant condition because, in fat (adipose) tissue, the circulating androgens are converted to an estrogen (estrone) which stimulates fibroid growth.

Premenopause

Premenopause or transitional years is that time later in the reproductive life cycle where again there is estrogen dominance and this increased estrogen environment triggers some mechanism to cause increased growth of uterine fibroids. It is also interesting that with the onset of menopause, a low estrogenic environment is present and many of these enlarged uterine fibroids will decrease in size (unless that woman goes on estrogen replacement therapy).

Presence of Hormone Disruptors

Finally, there are environmental factors, called hormone disruptors, which may act as hormones in the body or interfere with hormonal actions and cause the growth of uterine fibroids. Additionally eating foods with estrogens or estrogen like compounds are being associated with stimulation. DDT and other organic chemicals are examples of hormonal disruptors.

STRESS

Stress may be a factor which interferes with the normal pituitary-ovarian axis and therefore produces an estrogen dominant environment which can contribute to fibroid growth.

GENETIC FACTORS

Genetic patterns are presently being studied and hopefully will result in determining the cause of fibroid development. Studies currently being done indicate that there could be an error in the gene that controls the replication rate of uterine muscle tissue which give rise to fibroids.

TREATMENT OF FIBROIDS

If you have been diagnosed with having fibroids and they are not causing any symptoms, no treatment is probably necessary. Your physician will closely monitor them and you should inform him or her if symptoms appear. However, if your fibroids are causing symptoms, you need medical attention and you should decide on the several types of treatments (surgical or non-surgical) available to you.

I DO NOT WANT SURGERY, IS THERE ANYTHING ELSE?

Although surgery is a frightening thought to someone who has never had it, in some cases it is absolutely necessary. You are not responsible for what your body is doing in the formation of fibroids but you must consider all of the facts to alleviate this condition.

WHAT DETERMINES THE TYPE OF SURGICAL TREATMENT?

The type of surgery that a woman selects for removal of her fibroids depends on several factors such as:

- The size and number of the fibroids
- The location of the fibroids
- If she wishes to preserve her uterus
- If she wishes to become pregnant

TREATMENT DESIGN

The design of the treatment for fibroids is directed at the following:

- Removal of fibroids (surgical procedures)
- Shrinking the fibroids (drug treatment)
- Surgical shrinking of the fibroids (myolysis, uterine artery embolization

HELPING YOU MAKE YOUR DECISION: WHAT A PHYSICIAN SHOULD DO

The physician should inform the patient of all of her choices and provide enough information so that she can make a careful and intelligent decision. If the patient wishes to preserve her uterus, the physician should respect her wish. If the physician cannot perform the myomectomy operation with a high degree of expertise and precision, then he or she should refer the patient to a specialist with the requisite skill, expertise and experience. **DO NOT SETTLE FOR LESS!!!**

A PHILOSOPHY OF FIBROID MANAGEMENT

Management of a patient with fibroids is a philosophical consideration both for the patient and the physician. The main question is "what is the desire of the patient if she were symptomatic now"? If the patient prefers to salvage her uterus, then she should have that option and the treatment would be a uterine-sparing procedure. The consideration for the physician would then be, what is the best uterine-sparing procedure to do based on the size of the uterus and the symptoms presenting.

TREATMENT PROCEDURES: A QUICK OUTLINE

I. NON INVASIVE PROCEDURES

    A. MEDICAL TREATMENT

        1. HORMONES
             Oral contraceptives (not effective)
             Depo Provera
             Danocrine/lupron
             Mifeprex (antiprogesterone)

        2. DRUGS (investigative)– inhibit cell growth and proliferation
             Serums
             antigrowth factor
             retinoids

II. INVASIVE PROCEDURES

    A. OUTPATIENT SERVICES

        1. LAPAROSCOPIC PROCEDURES

            1. MYOMECTOMY
            2. MYOLYSIS

2.   HYSTEROSCOPIC MYOMECTOMY

3.   UTERINE ARTRY EMBOLIZATON

4.   ULTRASONIC

B.   INPATIENT SERVICES

1.   MYOMECTOMY
conventional
laser

2.   HYSTERECTOMY

SURGICAL TREATMENTS

REMOVAL OF FIBROIDS

THE HYSTERECTOMY

Let's begin with the more serious procedure—the hysterectomy. In this operation, there is a complete removal of the uterus with or without the removal of the ovaries. Now, this procedure offers the only complete cure because obviously, your uterus is removed. However, there is an alternative to this radical procedure called a **myomectomy** which removes only the fibroids. If you are advised to get a hysterectomy as the only choice for treating fibroids, get a second or third opinion, especially, if you have not yet had children or not through with childbearing or do not prefer to lose your uterus. Some women have experienced some sexual dysfunction following hysterectomy such as a change in their orgasmic response. Women who are aware of strong uterine contractions during orgasms notice that after hysterectomy, the quality of orgasm changes. This cannot be reversed.

TYPES OF HYSTERECTOMIES BASED ON PORTION OF UTERUS REMOVED

Complete or Total Hysterectomy

In this procedure, your entire uterus is removed.

Supracervical or Partial Hysterectomy

The top part of the uterus is removed but the lower part containing the cervix is left in place.

TYPES OF HYSTERECTOMIES BASED ON ROUTE OF REMOVAL

Abdominal Hysterectomy

In an abdominal hysterectomy, an incision is made through the abdominal wall and the uterus removed.

Vaginal Hysterectomy

A vaginal hysterectomy involves removing the uterus through the vagina. Usually, this procedure is performed when there is a prolapsed uterus (a uterus that has fallen from its usual position).

Laparoscopic Assisted Vaginal hysterectomy (LAVH)

The hysterectomy is performed with the assistance of the laparoscope.

THE MYOMECTOMY

If a woman wishes to retain her uterus and only have the fibroids removed, then by all means she should request a myomectomy. Myomectomy is a surgical procedure in which only the fibroids are removed from the uterus and the uterus is reconstructed to its normal state. Thus, because the uterus is left intact, the reproductive potential regarding childbearing is spared if this is an issue. Also, a woman may just want to keep her uterus for whatever reasons unique to her.

After myomectomy, all symptoms related to the fibroids should disappear and the uterus is able to perform its normal function of conception, pregnancy, and delivery. However, if pregnancy occurs the patient should have delivery by C-section. There are several surgical procedures that a fibroid can be removed and include the following:

TYPES OF MYOMECTOMY

Abdominal Myomectomy

An abdominal myomectomy also called a laparotomy involves making a horizontal or vertical incision in the abdomen, removing all of the fibroids and then surgically repairing the uterus. The myomectomy can be performed by conventional techniques or by laser or Harmonic scapel technique.

Hysteroscopic Myomectomy

In a hysteroscopic myomectomy, a thin telescope-like instrument called a **hysteroscope** is inserted through the vagina and cervix into the uterus and the fibroid(s) removed. This procedure has limitations in which only those fibroids that are found in the uterus cavity can be removed. It may be beneficial if this is the only fibroid(s) responsible for the symptoms.

Laparoscopic Myomectomy

A laparoscopic myomectomy consists of also inserting a telescope like instrument called a **laparoscope** through a small incision just below the navel where the physician can see inside the abdomen. The surgeon then uses very thin surgical tools to remove the fibroids. This procedure also has limitations in that it is useful for only a small number of fibroids. If multiple fibroids are present, most surgeons resort to the abdominal myomectomy approach.

WILL FIBROIDS RETURN AFTER A MYOMECTOMY?

Fibroids can return in a small percentage of cases in some women after a myomectomy. Why some women are prone to this recurrence is still a mystery. The biological mechanism(s) for growth of fibroids in certain women in the first place are responsible for possible reappearance.

MYOLYSIS

In this procedure a patient is initially given medications to shrink the fibroids and then, a laparoscopic procedure is performed in which an electrical needle cryoprobe or laser is used to destroy the fibroid tissue and blood vessels feeding those fibroids near the uterine surface.

FIBROIDS AND PREGNANCY

SHOULD A WOMAN HAVE A MYOMECTOMY DURING PREGNANCY?

Unless a fibroid(s) is causing major complications during pregnancy it is best to leave them alone.

HOW AM I TREATED IF I AM PREGNANT AND HAVE UNDERGONE A MYOMECTOMY?

A patient should have delivery by a C-section if she had a myomectomy.

OTHER PROCEDURES TO MANAGE FIBROIDS

UTERINE ARTERY EMBOLIZATION

This procedure is performed by a specialized physician known as an **interventional radiologist** in the radiology department of the hospital. This procedure involves making a small incision in the leg from which a catheter is carefully guided through the femoral artery (artery supplying blood to the leg) until it reaches the uterine artery which, is the major artery supplying blood to the uterus. Then, the catheter is used to inject tiny pellets into the small arteries feeding the fibroids. These pellets block the blood supply to fibroids and because of the subsequent blood deprivation, the fibroids degenerate and are reduced in size. This procedure is used to alleviate excessive bleeding associated with the fibroids.

TREATMENT OF FIBROIDS
WITH MEDICINES

DRUG TREATMENT FOR FIBROIDS

ARE THERE ANY DRUGS THAT WILL PREVENT OR ELIMINATE FIBROIDS?

No. Unfortunately, there are not any drugs at present that will prevent or eliminate fibroids. However, there are drugs that can shrink the size of fibroids but, they must be continually taken. The main drawback to taking these medications is when you stop taking them, the fibroids can re-grow to their original size. Also, because of the side effects of these drugs you can not take them continually for more than 6 months.

A BRIEF BACKGROUND ON DRUG ACTION

In order to understand the drug therapy for fibroids, it is necessary to provide some basic information on how drugs work. You will see terms like drug **analogs** and **agonists** such a GnRH agonists when discussing treatment for fibroids.

DRUG ANALOGS

A drug analog is simply a drug that looks very similar to a particular chemical in the body. In the case of hormones, a drug is designed to look like that hormone. The body does not know the difference—it thinks that the drug is actually the hormone. The principal is similar to the design of artificial sweeteners or products that "are not real butter".

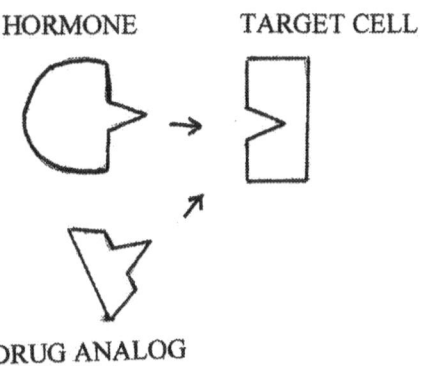

HORMONE   TARGET CELL

DRUG ANALOG

HOW HORMONE ANALOGS WORK

Recall that hormones bind to certain sites on target cells called receptors. Hormone analogs are synthetic chemicals that can also bind to these receptors.

DRUG AGONISTS VS DRUG ANTAGONISTS

An agonist binds to a receptor and **produces** a response. An antagonist binds to a receptor but no response is elicited. Thus, it **blocks** any response.

HORMONE THERAPY

Drug therapy such as hormone therapy is directed at components of the female reproductive system so it is important that you review the hormones of the female reproductive system.

MEDICATION TO SHRINK FIBROIDS

Gonadotropin-releasing hormone agonists (GnRH agonists)

These agents block the body from producing the female hormones estrogen and progesterone that cause the process of menstruation. When these drugs are administered they cause menopause to be temporarily induced and, as a consequence, the woman does not have her periods.

GnRH agonists include the following:

- Lupron (leuprolide acetate)
- Zoladex (goserelin acetate)
- Synarel (nafarelin acetate)

HOW DO GnRH AGONISTS WORK?

Without going into any detailed pharmacology, the GnRH agonists initially stimulates the pituitary to produced the gonadotropins FSH and LH. However, continued use of the GnRH agonists cause a suppression of FSH and LH hormones. When these hormones are not produced they are not available to act on the ovaries. So, the ovaries are basically turned off and no estrogen or progesterone is produced causing a menopausal like condition.

WHY PRESCRIBE GnRH AGONISTS?

The rationale for producing these drugs is to reduce the size of the fibroids prior to surgery to make them easier to remove. However, a down side to this treatment is that if some of the smaller fibroids are reduced further they could become small enough to be missed during surgery. It must be pointed out that in skilled and experienced physician hands, this pretreatment is unnecessary because all fibroids can be removed when performing a myomectomy. Therefore, there is not a need to reduce the size of the fibroids.

HORMONAL THERAPY IS TEMPORARY

There cannot be a prolonged course of hormonal therapy so any effects are temporary. Once you cease taking the drug, the fibroids will re-grow to their original size within 4 to 6 months.

SIDE EFFECTS OF GnRH THERAPY

Women who are taking these medications will experience symptoms such as vaginal dryness, hot flashes, night sweats and mood swings (menopausal symptoms).

THE WOMEN'S LASER INSTITUTE

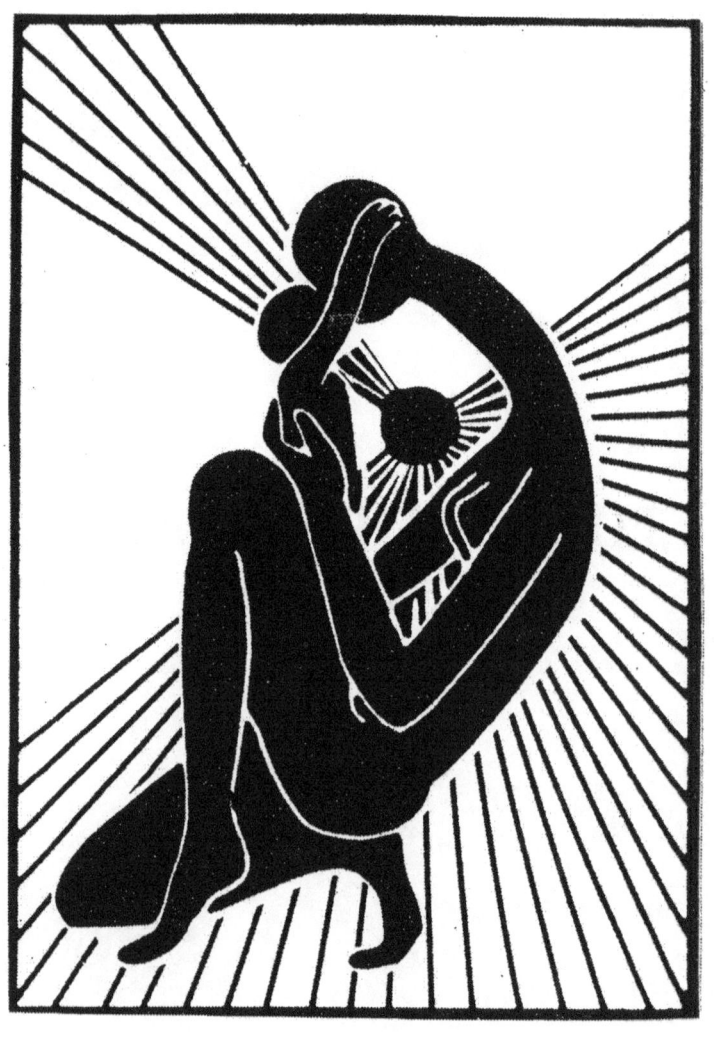

THE PHILOSOPHY

The philosophy of treatment management of fibroids at the Women's Laser Institute is that no woman should lose her uterus as a result of fibroid disease, unless there is no other option available or that the patient has been adequately informed and concurs in the decision.

The management of uterine fibroids is a philosophical approach. The philosophy of the physician should be, what is the best treatment for the patient, considering her desires and informed decision. The patient's philosophy should be what is the best treatment for me considering relief of symptoms, minimizing blood loss, prevention of pelvic adhesions and a chance for childbearing function, if desired. Other considerations would be cost, time in the hospital, and time away from work.

SUCCESS AT THE WOMEN'S LASER INSTITUTE

FAQs (Frequently Asked Questions) to Dr. Moorehead

1. How many operations (myomectomies) have you performed?

Approximately 800

2. How long have you been performing myomectomies?

I have been performing this surgery since 1983.

3. What is the most number of fibroids that you have removed from a single patient?

71

4. What is the smallest size fibroid that you have removed?

One which is the approximate size of a bb.

5. What is the largest size fibroid that you have removed?

One that weighed approximately 10 lbs (size of a watermelon)

6. How old was the youngest patient that you operated on to remove fibroids?

18 years of age

7. What age is the oldest patient that you have operated on to remove fibroids?

58 years of age

8. Has any of your myomectomy procedures turned into hysterectomies during the operation?

Only 3 out of approximately 800 operations.

9. Did any of your patients have to receive transfusions during the surgery?

Only 1 out of approximately 800 operations

10. How large does a fibroid have to be before it can be felt during a pelvic examination?

It depends on the location of the fibroid(s)

FIBROID TREATMENT RECOMMENDATIONS

The management of uterine fibroids is varied and even controversial. Our experience dictates that the management depends upon the size of the uterus, the symptoms present and the desire of the patient. If the uterus is less than 12 weeks size and there are no symptoms, then the patient can be followed without any treatment necessary. However, if the uterus is 12 weeks size or greater, the most important consideration is what is the desire of the patient? A uterus 12 weeks size or greater is a surgical problem and will require surgery unless a medical condition exists or patient refuses an invasive procedure. Also, what would be her preference if she were symptomatic now or in the future? If the patient preferred to salvage her uterus, regardless of her age or reproductive desire, she should have that option and her treatment should be accordingly. The choice would therefore be a myomectomy.

There are other treatments available but they are temporary methods at best. These treatments are listed as drug therapy, myolysis and even embolization. Because these treatment modalities are relatively recent in our practice the long term result is still unknown. There are several known factors that speak against these treatments as being definitive.

The first is that the uterus is a very vascular organ and there is a physiological mechanism by which the uterus repairs itself by generating new growth of blood vessels and blood supply. Thereby, over a period of time the uterus and the fibroid tissue would have recovery ability. Another factor is that the myometrial tissue (the tissue of fibroids) is made up with hormone receptor sites to estrogen progesterone and growth hormones.

With a regenerated blood supply, the remaining tissue of the fibroid will again undergo stimulation and regrowth. Lastly, the fibroids are often times numerous and multifaceted, therefore all areas may not respond or may respond differently.

THE CONSIDERATION OF MYOMECTOMY

Myomectomy should not be only considered as a surgical procedure. Consideration of myomectomy would be preoperative preparation, good operative technique, considering minimizing blood loss, prevention of pelvic adhesions, and postoperative management.

Minimally Invasive Surgery

Minimally invasive surgery such as laparoscopy or hysteroscopy should be considered as temporary solutions only. Even though these procedures are outpatient and less expensive, they can only remove fibroids that are visible or growing on the surface of the uterus (externally or internally). Therefore both procedures are limited to the fibroids that can be visualized and removed.

These procedures are for primary relief of symptoms, knowing that the fibroids may still remain within the walls of the uterus and by their growth over time, symptoms may recur.

Our experience over the past 20 years has dictated that the only way to remove all fibroids from the uterus, minimize blood loss and facilitate the prevention of adhesions is by laser/ultrasonic myomectomy.

Our experience has allowed us to refute many surgical precepts and institute new modalities, including expanded criteria for the preservation of a woman's reproductive organs, if she so desires. This consideration should be given regardless of age or reproductive desires. The greatest contribution as a physician is to educate the patient and encourage the patient to participate in the decision for the treatment recommended.

THE MYOMECTOMY AT THE WOMEN'S LASER INSTITUTE

A WALK THROUGH OF THE OPERATION

PREOPERATIVE TESTS

You will be scheduled to have pre-operative lab work performed. If any of your test are abnormal, we will inform you immediately and make the needed adjustments.

PREPARING FOR SURGERY

Your Surgery Date

You must inform us of the date that your menstrual cycle starts so that your surgery can be confirmed. It is also extremely important that you use protection against a pregnancy for this cycle.

Personal Items

You will be asked to please leave your rings and other jewelry at home. Bring a robe and slippers and night clothes (gowns) to wear when you no longer want to wear the hospital gown. Also, bring hair necessities, toothbrush, toothpaste, and body lotion.

Medicines

Do not take medicines such as aspirin, bufferin, Advil or Motrin for 10 days prior to your surgery date.

The Night Before Your Surgery

The night before surgery, you will be given fasting instructions and an enema.

THE OPERATION

The morning of the operation

We usually schedule surgeries at 7:00 am. The patient is usually awakened around 5:00 am and instructed to shower and douche. Afterward she is wheeled to the preoperative area where the nurses and anesthesiologist prep her for surgery.

After the patient is anesthetized, a catheter is introduced. The surgery begins with an incision on the abdomen.

HOSPITAL STAY AFTER SURGERY

Myomectomy requires a two (2) day hospital stay and the patient can return to her work activities as early as 2-3 weeks.

POST-OPERATIVE CARE AND INSTRUCTIONS

First 24 Hours

The first 24 hours after surgery is essential to the patient's recovery. When the patient stands, she should make every effort to stand erect (the incision will not be harmed). Also, good body movement will help expedite recovery.

Another important step is to cough. This will help prevent pneumonia. The patient may find it necessary to place a pillow on her stomach as a support.

FOOD

A light, clear diet is served on the first surgical day. When the patient is able to eat a regular meal, she should request only broiled, baked or steamed foods. Fried, greasy and highly seasoned foods should be avoided at all times.

WALKING

To get rid of gaseous pockets that form after major surgery, the patient will need to walk as much as possible. She should never walk if she feels weak, and during her walks she should take rest breaks in-between. Unless and until she is comfortable, she should walk with assistance.

BATHING

If at all possible, a shower should be taken the day after surgery – with assistance. This will feel refreshing, along with fresh linens and bed clothes.

The patient should not rub her incision; it should be gently patted dry.

POST-OPERATIVE INSTRUCTIONS

GOING HOME

The patient should arrange in advance to have someone drive her home from the hospital. Because the trip may tire her, she should plan to rest for the remainder of the day. Our office should be contacted to arrange a post-op visit for 2 weeks after discharge.

ACTIVITIES

During the six weeks period following her surgery, the patient will experience peaks and valleys in the way she feels. She should not let a "bad" day get her down; she will probably feel better the next day.

A good rule is that activity during the first week at home should not be any more than that allowed on the last day of your hospital stay. The patient is encouraged to gradually increase her activity for progressively longer periods of time. Whenever desired, it is permissible to take showers, or even wash the hair. In fact, sometimes these things can really make the patient feel better. Good days may be associated with more activity and bad days should be associated with more rest.

WALKS

Depending on the condition of the patient, she should try to take a short walk (in the house) each day. If she should tire, she should stop and rest.

STAIRS

During the first week, the number of trips up and down stairs should be limited. As the patient feels stronger, she may increase stair climbing as she wishes.

RECOVERY TIMETABLE

First & Second Week:

Frequent rest periods.

Third Week:

The patient may prepare a light meal and perform light housekeeping chores. She should plan at least two rest periods each day and may gradually increase activities, take short rides, increase walking, go shopping, and increase social activities.

Fourth through Sixth Week:

Return to normal activities at home and work (in most cases). However, strenuous activities should not be resumed until 4 to 6 weeks after surgery. The patient is not permitted to drive until advised by physician.

MARITAL RELATIONS

Normal sexual activities should not be resumed until after the four to six week post-operative check-up. This will allow ample time to heal.

CARE OF INCISION

Although the incision may appear somewhat healed by the time the patient is discharged, the healing process actually continues for several weeks.

The steri strips or bandages that may have been placed on the incision can be left on until they come off by themselves or until the patient finds them annoying. The sutures are absorbed and do not have to be removed. If the incision should become wet, it should be carefully dried by patting. The incision may bleed lightly or drain a bit for several weeks after surgery. This is not a cause for alarm. Simply clean the incision with salt water compresses and cover with a clean, dry dressing.

However, if the area should become red, tender, or drain excessively, our office should be contacted immediately.

DIET

A well-balanced diet high in vitamin C and protein is important in the healing process. Additionally, a good diet can promote regular bowel and bladder habits. Although the patient may eat virtually anything she wishes, she should try to include roughage in her diet and drink six to eight glasses of water per day. It is not wise to try to diet for weight loss during convalescence.

BLADDER CARE

Gynecological surgery patients have a catheter inserted at the time of surgery. Once the catheter is removed, it may take a while for the bladder to return to normal functions. It is very possible to have bladder spasms or pain after gynecological surgery. It is not possible to have a catheter without running a low grade infection. These problems are most often alleviated with medication.

The patient should contact the office if she experiences any unusual bladder symptoms.

VAGINAL DISCHARGE

Slight discharge or spotting is normal in the first few weeks after surgery. The patient may be given a special vaginal cream to insert each evening. She should not douche unless specifically instructed to do so.

If at any time, the bleeding becomes profuse or bright red, contact the office at once.

PROBLEMS

The patient should telephone the doctor/nurse if any of the following problems occur:

- Burning or pressure during urination
- Bright red bleeding from the vagina
- Swelling, tenderness, redness around the incision
- Chills, fever, or severe headache
- Fainting or constant dizziness
- Severe cramping
- Pain which cannot be alleviated with Tylenol
- Any other unexplained pains or problems

PHILOSOPHY, SUMMARY AND RECOMMENDATIONS

Learning about the reproductive system and uterine function, preparation has been made for the understanding of uterine disease and management.

Additionally, it is important to learn about management and treatment options. Knowing that uterine fibroids are benign tumors the principal consideration would be how to achieve the highest quality of life. Would the option be a decision for a uterine sparing procedure or consideration for a hysterectomy? Hysterectomy is a viable treatment option, but knowingly, not the only option.

Once the diagnosis of uterine fibroids has been made, the next consideration is that of management. There is an array of treatment options which allow for the retention of the uterus. The options are based on the treatment of symptoms versus treating the fibroids.

The first consideration in treating the symptoms is medical management. Unfortunately, there are no medications to prevent fibroids or permanently shrink them. The purpose of medical treatment is primarily two-fold, to relieve symptoms, i.e.- to control the bleeding associated with the fibroids, and reduction in discomfort; or to shrink the size of the fibroids to facilitate the surgical procedure.

The medications available for this use are:

- Oral contraceptives
- Depo-Provera
- Danocrine
- Lupron (GNRH)
- Mifepristone (antiprogesterone)

All of these agents function by altering the estrogen environment around the fibroids. By preventing an estrogen dominant environment (menopause) the fibroids undergo a reduction in size. Side affects from this condition could be menopausal symptoms, hot flashes, night sweats and more importantly accelerated bone loss. Unfortunately, fibroids return to pretreatment size very rapidly upon discontinuance of the medication. An additional drawback to medical suppression is that the small fibroids present may also undergo change which could make them impossible to palpate and remove during a myomectomy. This would lead to a "false recurrence" when in fact they were not removed at the time of myomectomy.

Unless all fibroids are removed at the time of myomectomy, it is not possible to calculate a true recurrence rate. There are other investigative drugs under study, but so far there is no medical approach beyond that which has been discussed.

The surgical or invasive treatments are divided into minor surgical approach and major surgery.

Minor surgery:

- Laparoscopic myolysis
- Laparoscopic myomectomy
- Hysteroscopic myomectomy
- Uterine Artery Embolization

Improvements in endoscopic technology has allowed for the laparoscopic or hysteroscopic approach for myomectomy. Hysteroscopy is the insertion of a small telescope through the cervix into the uterine cavity. The submucus fibroid is visualized and removed by electrical dissection. This procedure is performed as outpatient surgery and has been a major advance in the treatment of fibroids in the uterine cavity. The limitations of this procedure is only the fibroids in the cavity can be removed and therefore, if other fibroids exist in the uterus, they will remain intact.

Laparoscopic myomectomy is another way to remove fibroids surgically. Again, this is outpatient surgery although it may require an overnight stay. The laparoscope is a small telescope introduced through a small incision in the navel. The pedunculated, serosal or superficial intramural fibroids are the only ones to be removed. The surgery is lengthy and sometimes technically difficult. The closures of the uterine incisions are difficult by the laparoscopic approach and should be performed only by a skilled endoscopic surgeon. Since this closure of the incision is technically difficult there has been reports of spontaneous uterine rupture. Again only the clearly obvious fibroids can be removed.

Myolysis is a procedure also done through the laparoscope. This procedure shrinks fibroids without removing them, thereby relieving the symptoms. This procedure is accomplished by inserting a probe or needle into the fibroid and destroying the tissue by electrical current, laser vaporization, or freezing technique with a cryoprobe. By this destruction of tissue, the blood supply is compromised and tissue necrosis occurs resulting in shrinkage of the fibroid. This necrosis of tissue may cause significant pain and scar tissue formation. As true with the endoscopic procedures, only the fibroids visualized can be treated.

Uterine artery embolization is a procedure done to reduce the size of fibroids by compromising the blood supply to the uterus. This procedure is performed by a Radiologist who specializes in using catheters and x-ray imaging to reach remote sites. In this case, a catheter is positioned into the uterine artery and tiny pellets are injected. These particles produce blockage in the small arteries of the uterus and around the fibroids. Deprived of a blood supply the fibroids undergo necrosis and over time shrink in size. Most patients experience intense pain and require pain medication. Some may require readmission for pain management. This procedure is done for patients with heavy bleeding and anemia. The long-term result of this procedure is uncertain, but the uterus has the capacity to revascularize the area and this could stimulate the regrowth of fibroids.

Major surgery:

Major surgery options are abdominal myomectomy (conventional, laser) and hysterectomy. Myomec-tomy can be performed by conventional techniques or by laser, or Harmonic scalpel technique. The goal of myomectomy should be to remove all of the fibroids that can be identified with the least amount of bleeding and injury to the reproductive tract. The uterus is well vascularized and therefore significant intraoperative bleeding is frequently encountered. The result of excessive blood loss and tissue trauma give rise to adhesion formation that could compromise a woman's fertility. It is therefore most important to have a skilled surgeon perform the myomectomy.

Conventional myomectomy is performed using the customary instruments. This procedure is complicated by excessive bleeding and frequently the procedure is abandoned before all fibroids can be removed. As a result there is an increased risk of blood transfusion and postoperative adhesion formation.

Laser myomectomy or myomectomy performed with the Harmonic scalpel are procedures that require additional training and skill. However, the added advantage of using this technology is that blood loss is minimized and tissue trauma is also reduced. The function of these surgical tools is that as the instrument is used the heat manifested by their action seals, small blood vessels as it cuts, thereby minimizing the blood loss and permitting the surgeon to remove all fibroids detected and less risk of post operative adhesions. By these methods the risk of blood transformation, adhesion formation and compromised fertility is drastically reduced.

Hysterectomy is the removal of the uterus and thereby the fibroids as a part of the uterus are also eliminated. However, by removing the uterus, reproductive potential is eliminated as well as the presenting symptoms and thereby the risk of recurrence of fibroids is zero.

Most women do not wish to lose their reproductive organs whether or not they are interested in childbearing function. The desire to not lose the uterus should be honored by the gynecologist and uterine sparing procedures should be advocated. No woman should be subjected to a hysterectomy because of fibroids unless she has been fully informed about the alternative and agrees to the decision.

If the decision is made to have a hysterectomy, then based on size of the fibroids in the uterus, medical history of the patient and previous surgical history if any, the type of procedure would be determined. Also, depending on the age and desire of the patient a consideration is made as to the removal of the ovaries.

The decision to have a hysterectomy should be based on benefits and or risks to the patient. The surgical approach can be tailored to presenting conditions; i.e.-abdominal hysterectomy, vaginal hysterectomy, and laparoscopic assisted vaginal hysterectomy (LAVH). This is determined by the skill and experience of the surgeon as well as the indications of the problem. Because of the potential risk and possible complications the patient should be well informed prior to the procedure and aware of the alternatives available.

Any surgical procedure has the risk of postoperative adhesion formation. In patients that want to preserve their childbearing functions by selecting a uterine-sparing procedure, post operative adhesions are the greatest risk towards compromising their fertility. Myomectomy has a direct tendency toward post operative ahesions and techniques to prevent the development should be followed.

EMPOWERING YOURSELF

TAKE CHARGE

QUESTIONS YOU SHOULD ASK YOURSELF

1. Do I desire to become pregnant?
2. Do I want to keep my uterus
3. Do I want to be surgically cured of fibroids with a hysterectomy (first and final surgery)

Questions You should ask your Doctor?

1. How many myomectomies have you performed?
2. What is your success rate?

MAKE THE RIGHT DECISION FOR YOU

We hope that this book has provided enough information so that you are able to make the right decision for your treatment of fibroids.

CHECKLIST

DID YOU

- UNDERSTAND ALL OF THE INFORMATION YOU READ?
- READ ALL OF THE INFORMATION THAT YOU COULD ON FIBROIDS?
- ASK YOUR DOCTOR ALL OF THE PERTINENT QUESTIONS?
- FIND THE MOST EXPERIENCED SURGEON TO PERFORM THE OPERATION?

REFERENCES AND RESOURCES

There are numerous references and resource material regarding fibroids. Some are pamphlets, booklets, web information, books as well as very technical information. We have listed only a few.

1. Uterine fibroids. Pamphlet. The American College of Obstetricians and Gynecologists.

2. Fibroids: A Guide for Woman. 1996. Booklet. Andrew J. Friedman. The Health Information Network. HIN, Inc.

3. Common Uterine Conditions. Booklet. Agency for Health Care Policy and Research (AHCPR)/US Department of Health & Human Services.

4. What Every Black Woman Should Know About Fibroid Tumors. 1998. Nicole Walker. Ebony

5. No More Hysterectomies. 1989. Vicki Hufnagel. Plume Book

A PICTORIAL GALLERY OF FIBROIDS

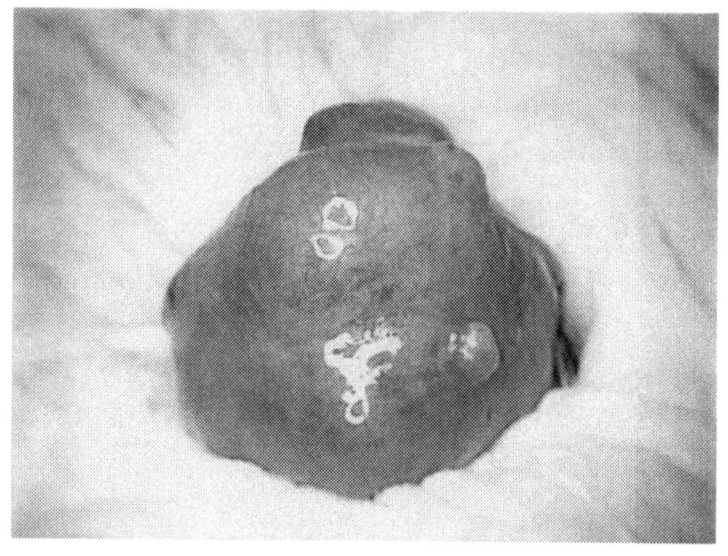

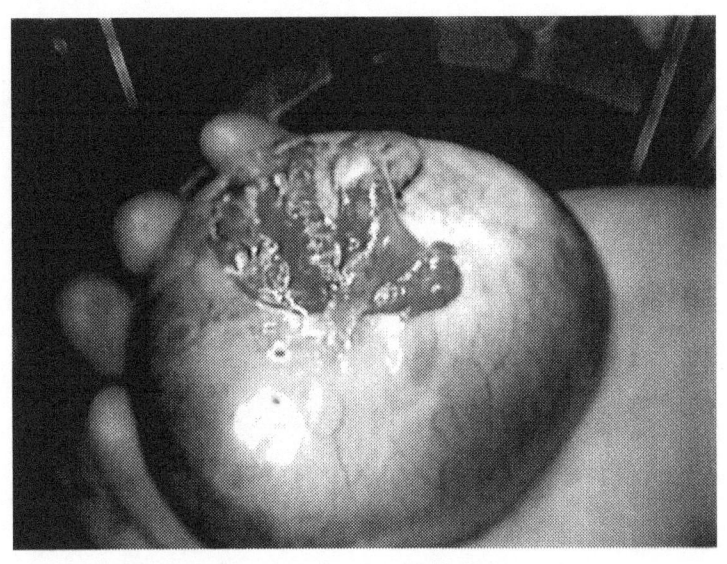

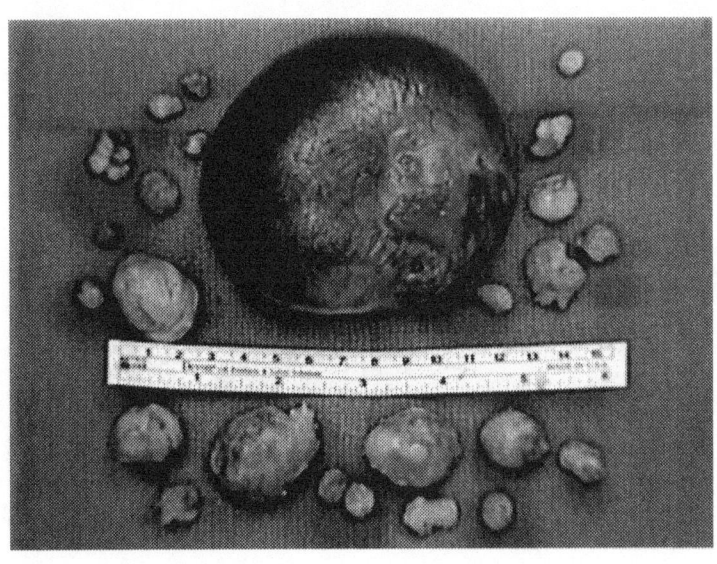

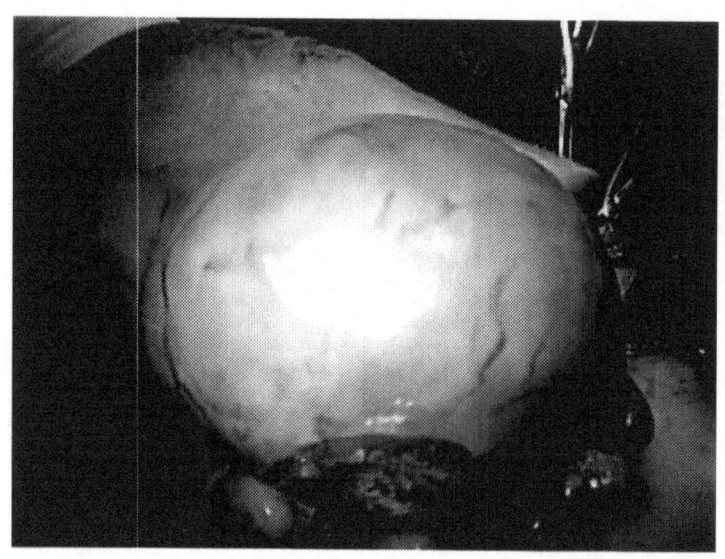

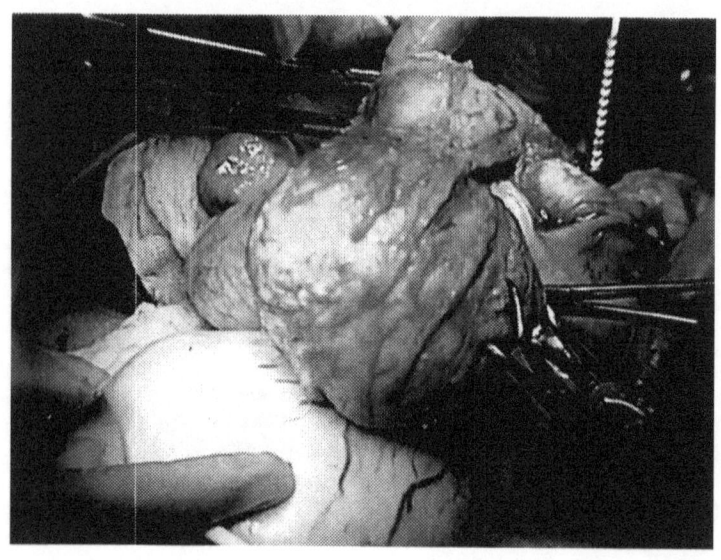

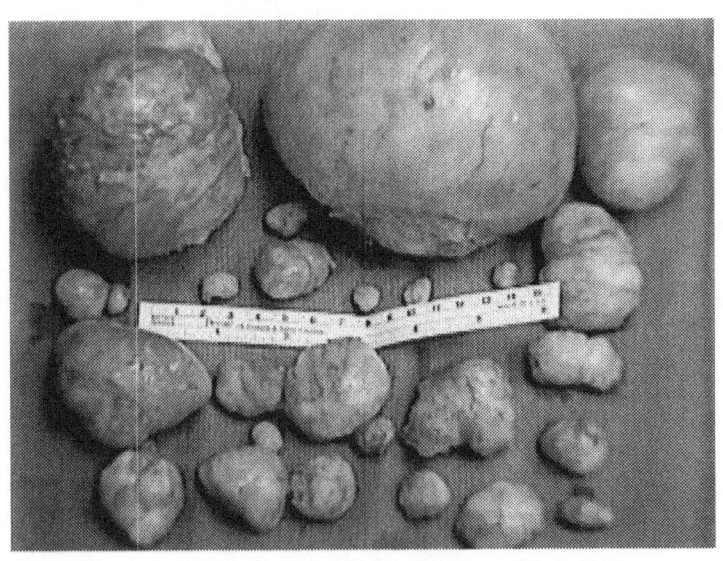

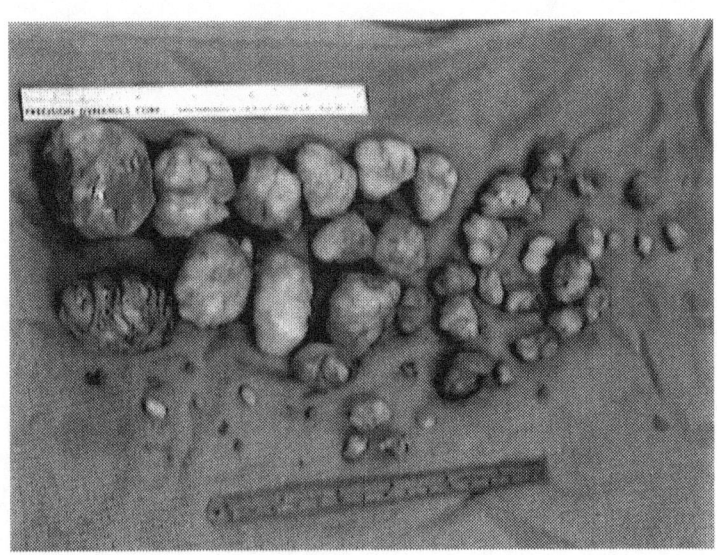

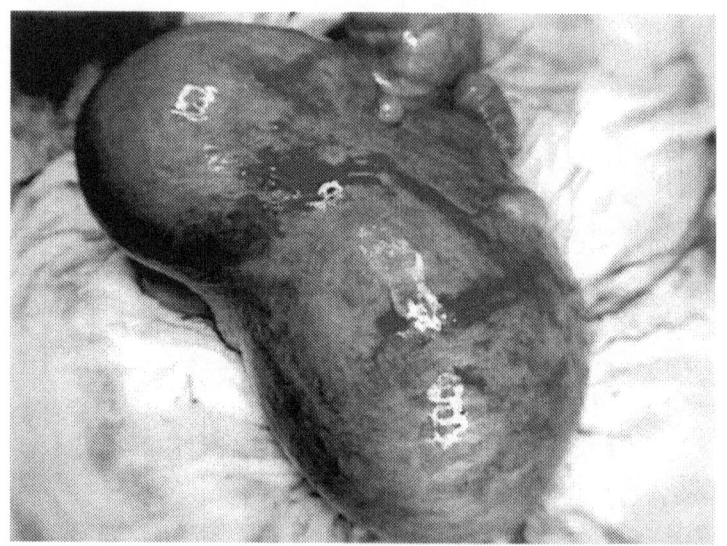

ABOUT THE AUTHORS

Dr. Myron Moorehead

Dr. Myron Moorehead received his M.D. from Meharry Medical College in Nashville, Tennessee, and served his internship at St. Joseph's Hospital in Syracuse, New York. He completed his residency training in Obstetrics and Gynecology at Walter Reed General Hospital in Washington, D.C. He began his private practice in Obstetrics and Gynecology in 1970.

Dr. Moorehead is the Director of the Women's Laser Institute in New Orleans, Louisiana and is also a clinical Assistant Professor in the Dept. of Obstetrics and Gynecology Tulane University School of Medicine

He is a member of the American Society for Reproductive Medicine, the Gynecological Laser Society and the Society of Reproductive Surgeons. He is certified by the American Board of Obstetrics and Gynecology and is a fellow of the American College of Obstetrics and Gynecologists. Dr.

Moorehead, the recipient of numerous awards has performed approximately 800 myomectomies for fibroid tumors.

Dr. Bryan Lewis

Bryan Lewis, Ph.D. is a Professor of Microbiology and the author of several books on Microbiology and Chemistry. He became aware of Dr. Moorehead and the Women's Laser Institute when his wife was seeking surgical treatment for her fibroid tumors. Dr. Moorehead provided a successful alternative (myomectomy) for fibroid removal other than hysterectomy. Dr. & Mrs. Lewis believe that more women should be exposed to alternatives to hysterectomy for fibroid removal after she was a recipient of this kind of surgery.